BELL'S PALSY MANAGEMENT DIET COOKBOOK

Discover Nourishing Recipes And Lifestyle Tips: Empowering Recovery Through Nutritious Choices-Effective Strategies For Healing And Well-Being

DR. SHAYLA LEWIS

Table of Contents

DISCLAIMER

Write a brief complete Disclaimer for my diet cook book telling them that the author is not in any association with any company, business or individual and also this book is written by the authors knowledge and understanding

The information provided in this diet cookbook is based on the author's personal knowledge and understanding. The author is not affiliated with, endorsed by, or associated with any company, business, or individual. The recipes and dietary advice contained within this book are intended for informational purposes only. Readers should consult with a healthcare professional or a registered dietitian before making any significant changes to their diet or lifestyle. The author assumes no responsibility for any adverse effects that may result from the use or misuse of the information contained in this book.

CHAPTER ONE

Understanding Bell's Palsy

Bell's palsy is a disorder characterized by abrupt weakness or paralysis on one side of the face as a result of inflammation or facial nerve injury. Symptoms may include drooping of the lips, trouble shutting the eye, and loss of facial expressions on the affected side. Understanding these symptoms can aid in early detection and treatment, which typically includes medications, physical therapy, and dietary changes to promote nerve health and recovery.

Importance of Nutrition: How Food Influences Healing

Nutrition is critical in the treatment of Bell's Palsy because it provides important nutrients that reduce inflammation and promote nerve regeneration. Consuming foods high in vitamins B12, B6, and D, as well as antioxidants such as vitamins C and E, can aid with neuron function and repair. Consuming anti-inflammatory foods like leafy greens, berries, and fatty fish can also help to alleviate symptoms and speed up recovery.

The fundamentals of low-carb, antioxidant-rich, and anti-inflammatory diets.

A low-carb diet promotes steady blood sugar levels, which is good for nerve function. Antioxidant-rich meals shield nerve cells from injury by neutralizing free radicals, whilst anti-inflammatory foods alleviate inflammation and pain linked with Bell's palsy. Consume plenty of veggies, lean proteins, healthy fats, and whole grains, but avoid processed foods, sugary snacks, and trans fats.

Navigating the Cookbook: Tips for Success

To effectively navigate Bell's Palsy Management Diet Cookbook, begin by familiarising yourself with the major ingredients and recipes that follow the prescribed dietary criteria. Plan your meals ahead of time and create a shopping list to ensure you have all of the supplies. Try making meals in batches to save time and keep your diet consistent. Use the cookbook's recommendations and adaptations to keep your meals interesting and on track with your dietary objectives.

Adopting a Healthier Lifestyle Beyond Bell's Palsy Management

Adopting a healthier lifestyle entails more than simply nutritional adjustments; it also requires regular physical activity, appropriate sleep, stress management, and staying hydrated. Incorporate mild workouts, such as yoga or walking, to promote circulation and overall health. Practice mindfulness or meditation to minimize stress, which can have a bad impact on nerve health. Adopting these holistic ways will help you recover from Bell's palsy and enhance your overall health.

What is Bell's palsy?

Bell's Palsy is characterized by abrupt and temporary weakening or paralysis of the muscles on one side of the face. It happens when the facial nerve, which controls the facial muscles, gets irritated or compressed. This disorder can cause one side of your face to droop, making it difficult to close your eyes or smile from that side. Understanding Bell's Palsy requires acknowledging that it is typically transitory and not life-threatening, with most people recovering completely within a few months.

Causes and Risk Factors

The actual etiology of Bell's Palsy is unknown, but it is thought to be associated with viral infections like herpes simplex, which causes cold sores. Other risk factors include diabetes, upper respiratory infections, and a family history of the disease. Stress and damaged immune systems might also raise vulnerability. Identifying these risk factors can aid in early discovery and rapid treatment to avoid serious problems.

Signs and Symptoms

Bell's Palsy symptoms often arise suddenly and include drooping on one side of the face, drooling, loss of taste on the front two-thirds of the tongue, heightened sensitivity to sound in one ear, and trouble shutting the afflicted eye. Recognizing these symptoms early on is critical for obtaining timely medical attention and initiating appropriate treatment to improve recovery.

Diagnostic and Treatment Options

The diagnosis of Bell's Palsy is mostly clinical, based on the patient's medical history and physical examination. To rule out other illnesses, doctors may use imaging tests such as an MRI or CT scan. Corticosteroids are commonly used to decrease inflammation, as well as antiviral treatments if a viral infection is detected. Physical therapy and face exercises are recommended for increasing muscular strength and coordination. Early intervention considerably improves the odds of complete recovery.

Importance of Diet in Management

A well-balanced diet is essential for managing Bell's Palsy since it promotes general health and helps with rehabilitation. Including foods high in vitamins B12, B6, and C, such as leafy greens, citrus fruits, and lean meats, can aid with nerve repair and immunological function. Staying hydrated and avoiding sugary and processed meals can help to reduce inflammation and promote recovery.

How Nutrition Impacts Healing

Nutrition is critical to the healing process because it provides the body with the resources it needs to repair and renew tissues. Proper eating can enhance the immune system, minimize inflammation, and speed up healing. A diet high in vitamins, minerals, and antioxidants can assist people with Bell's Palsy in maintaining their nerve function and overall health. Incorporating a range of fruits, vegetables, lean proteins, and whole grains ensures that the body receives a balanced amount of nutrients, which aids in healing.

Balanced eating entails ingesting a varied range of meals in the proper amounts to supply the body with all of the necessary nutrients it requires. This entails including carbohydrates, proteins, fats, vitamins, and minerals in your regular diet. A balanced diet is essential for someone with Bell's Palsy since it promotes general health and aids in the recovery of nerve function. Ensuring that each meal has a variety of these nutrients can assist sustain energy levels, support metabolic activities, and improve the body's ability to heal itself.

The role of macronutrients and micronutrients

Macronutrients—carbohydrates, proteins, and fats—provide the majority of energy and are required for biological activities and tissue repair. Micronutrients, such as vitamins and minerals, are also essential for good health, but in lesser amounts. Appropriate protein consumption aids muscle healing in Bell's Palsy patients, whereas healthy fats promote nerve cell integrity. Vitamins B12 and D, as well as minerals magnesium and zinc, are essential for nervous system health and function. Including a variety of nutrient-dense foods ensures that macronutrient and micronutrient requirements are met.

Effects of Diet on Nerve Health

Diet has a substantial impact on nerve health, with specific nutrients being especially useful for neuron function and repair.

Fish and flaxseed contain omega-3 fatty acids, which strengthen nerve cell membranes and prevent inflammation. Antioxidants included in berries and leafy greens protect nerves from oxidative stress.

Additionally, vitamins such as B-complex, particularly B1, B6, and B12, are essential for nerve function. Incorporating these nutrient-dense foods into your diet will help control and even relieve Bell's Palsy

Addressing Nutritional Deficits

Identifying and treating nutritional deficiencies is critical for patients with Bell's Palsy, as shortages in specific vitamins and minerals can increase symptoms. Vitamin B12, vitamin D, and magnesium are all common deficiencies that have an impact on nerve function. To treat this, a diet rich in varied food groups is required. Consuming dairy products, fortified cereals, and leafy greens, for example, can increase calcium and magnesium levels, whereas fish, eggs, and fortified milk can increase vitamin D intake. If dietary changes are insufficient, healthcare practitioners may offer supplements to help maintain optimal nutritional levels.

CHAPTER TWO

Exploring Low-Carb Diets

Low-carb diets aim to reduce carbohydrate intake while increasing protein and fat consumption. This method helps regulate blood sugar levels and may be useful for managing illnesses such as Bell's palsy by lowering inflammation. Understanding macronutrient balance is essential: seek to receive your energy from proteins like chicken, fish, and eggs, as well as healthy fats from avocados and almonds, while limiting your intake of bread, pasta, and sweets.

Benefits of Bell's Palsy Management

Adopting a low-carb diet can help with Bell's Palsy management by improving general neurological health and reducing inflammation, which is essential for nerve regeneration. The diet's concentration of nutrient-dense meals delivers important vitamins and minerals, which promote greater immune function and may speed up the healing process. This diet promotes recovery by stabilizing blood sugar levels and maintaining consistent energy levels.

Examples of Low-Carb Foods

Include a variety of low-carb meals in your diet to guarantee proper nourishment. Choose veggies with minimal carbohydrates but high vitamin content, such as spinach, broccoli, and bell peppers. Choose lean proteins like fish, chicken, and tofu, as well as healthy fats from olive oil, nuts, and seeds. Avoid high-carb foods like bread, pasta, rice, and sugary snacks in favor of low-carb alternatives such as cauliflower rice and zucchini noodles.

Practical Ideas for Low-Carb Cooking

With a few practical suggestions, you can make low-carb meals that are both easy and delicious. Begin by equipping your kitchen with low-carb staples such as fresh veggies, lean protein, and healthy fats. Use herbs and spices to enhance flavor without adding carbohydrates. Experiment with cooking methods such as grilling, baking, and sautéing to improve the flavor and texture of your meals. Preparing meals in bulk and repurposing leftovers can also help you save time and have a low-carb choice on hand at all times.

Low-Carb Meal Plan

Effective low-carb meal planning entails preparing a variety of recipes that are simple to prepare and delicious to consume. Begin by planning your meals for the week, including a variety of meats, vegetables, and healthy fats. Breakfast may be a veggie omelet with avocado, lunch a chicken salad with olive oil dressing, and dinner grilled salmon with steamed broccoli. Snack alternatives include almonds, cheese, and sliced vegetables with hummus. Planning ahead keeps you on track and makes food shopping easier.

Understanding Antioxidants

Antioxidants are chemicals that battle free radicals in your body and prevent cell damage. They protect nerve cells from oxidative stress, which can exacerbate Bell's Palsy symptoms. Antioxidants in your diet assist support the body's natural healing processes, resulting in faster recovery and improved general health.

Important for Nerve Health

Antioxidants are essential for persons with Bell's Palsy because they reduce inflammation and promote nerve regeneration. They help protect the facial nerves from additional damage and alleviate the severity of symptoms. Consuming antioxidant-rich foods regularly can assist your nervous system function and stay healthy.

Include foods that are high in antioxidants. Berries, dark leafy greens, nuts, seeds, and citrus fruits can all help you get more antioxidants in your diet. These foods are high in vitamins C and E, flavonoids, and polyphenols, all of which are potent antioxidants that promote nerve health and recovery.

Recipes Packed With Antioxidants

Incorporate antioxidant-rich ingredients into your meals to make them both delicious and nutritious. A spinach and berry smoothie, a mixed green salad with citrus dressing, or a quinoa and vegetable stir-fry can all give a good source of antioxidants. These dishes are simple to prepare and incorporate into your daily diet plan, ensuring that you obtain a balanced intake of these essential nutrients.

Incorporating Antioxidants Daily

To incorporate antioxidants into your daily diet, start with a fruit smoothie or a handful of nuts for breakfast. Snack on fruits like oranges or apples, and incorporate a variety of veggies into your lunch and dinner. Simple changes, such as using olive oil in cooking and adding spices like turmeric and ginger, can easily increase your antioxidant consumption.

Basics of Inflammation

Inflammation is the body's normal response to damage or illness, but chronic inflammation can worsen disorders such as Bell's Palsy. To effectively manage inflammation, incorporate meals high in antioxidants and omega-3 fatty acids, which help lower inflammatory indicators in the body. Understanding the various types of inflammation and their triggers can help guide dietary choices to reduce flare-ups and promote overall nerve health.

Effects on Bell's Palsy Symptoms

Chronic inflammation can exacerbate Bell's Palsy symptoms by causing facial nerve irritation and delaying recovery. Reducing inflammation through nutrition can help with pain relief, muscle function, and recovery. Individuals can improve their quality of life and control their symptoms by eating anti-inflammatory foods regularly and avoiding those that cause inflammation.

Anti-inflammatory foods to prioritize

Include fatty fish (salmon, mackerel), leafy greens (spinach, kale), nuts (almonds, walnuts), and berries (blueberries, strawberries) in your daily diet. These foods are abundant in antioxidants, vitamins, and omega-3 fatty acids, all of which help to combat inflammation. Furthermore, spices such as turmeric and ginger can give anti-inflammatory properties, making meals more nutritious and tasty.

Cooking Techniques to Reduce Inflammation
Choose cooking methods that maintain the nutritious value of your ingredients, such as steaming, grilling, or roasting. Deep-frying and excessive oil use should be avoided, as these can introduce inflammatory chemicals. Using olive oil or coconut oil sparingly and integrating fresh herbs and spices can improve flavor while preserving anti-inflammatory characteristics in your food.

Combine colorful veggies, lean proteins, and healthy fats to make well-balanced anti-inflammatory meals. For example, a meal could feature grilled fish, quinoa and kale salad, and roasted sweet potatoes. This strategy guarantees that you get a variety of nutrients and antioxidants, which assist in reducing inflammation and promote general health.

Importance of Meal Planning

Meal planning is essential for controlling Bell's Palsy because it ensures a balanced diet of nutrients that promote nerve health and rehabilitation. Meal planning allows you to focus on foods high in vitamins B12 and B6, omega-3 fatty acids, and antioxidants, all of which are necessary for nerve healing and overall health. This method decreases stress, eliminates the temptation for unhealthy snacking, and aids in the maintenance of a constant meal schedule, which is critical for people suffering from the fatigue and energy changes associated with Bell's Palsy.

Tips for Effective Meal Prep

Efficient meal preparation starts with choosing recipes that can be readily batch-cooked and stored. Begin by cutting vegetables, cooking grains, and preparing proteins in large quantities over the weekend. Use containers to portion meals for the week, ensuring quick and easy access. To minimize confusion, label each container with its date and contents. To make meals interesting, use a variety of textures and flavors, and keep a few quick-to-assemble snacks on hand, such as pre-cut fruit or mixed nuts, to keep you nourished throughout the day.

A nutrient-dense breakfast of a spinach and mushroom omelet with a side of whole grain toast is one example of a Bell's Palsy management diet plan. For lunch, make a quinoa salad with mixed greens, cherry tomatoes, avocado, and grilled chicken. Dinner might include salmon fillets with roasted sweet potatoes and steamed broccoli. Snacks could include Greek yogurt with berries or a handful of walnuts. Each meal and snack should include foods that promote nerve health, such as leafy greens, lean proteins, and healthy fats.

Adapting Recipes to Personal Preference

Consider dietary limitations, favorite flavors, and textures when customizing dishes. If a dish asks for a fish you don't like, substitute another that you do, such as tilapia instead of salmon. Vegetarians can replace meat with plant-based proteins like lentils or tofu. Adjust the seasoning amounts to your liking, and experiment with herbs and spices to make the dish more appetizing. The idea is to keep the nutritional value while keeping the meals pleasurable and customized to your preferences.

CHAPTER THREE

Shopping list and pantry staples

Creating a precise shopping list streamlines supermarket excursions and ensures that you have all of the necessary components. Whole grains such as quinoa and brown rice, canned beans, almonds, seeds, olive oil, and a variety of herbs and spices are must-have pantry mainstays for a Bell's Palsy diet.

Fresh vegetables such as leafy greens, avocados, berries, and citrus fruits should be available regularly. Having a well-organized pantry with these things makes it easy to cook healthful meals and adjust to any recipe adjustments or preferences you may have.

Importance of Beginning the Day Right

Starting your day with a good meal is essential for managing Bell's Palsy since it boosts your metabolism, offers energy, and promotes general health. A well-balanced meal helps boost concentration, regulate blood sugar levels, and alleviate morning weariness. To guarantee consistent energy throughout the morning, prioritize protein, healthy fats, and complex carbohydrates.

Quick and Easy Breakfast Recipes

Quick and easy breakfast ideas come in handy for individuals who have hectic mornings. Consider avocado toast with whole grain bread, overnight oats with chia seeds, or a vegetarian omelet. These meals may be prepared in about 15 minutes, allowing you to avoid skipping breakfast while still providing critical nutrients for neurological health and overall wellness.

Nutrient-Dense Smoothies and Shakes

Smoothies and shakes are ideal for a nutrient-dense breakfast to go. Blend spinach, berries, protein powder, flax seeds, and almond milk. This combination contains antioxidants, fiber, protein, and omega-3 fatty acids, all of which promote nerve function and overall health. To add variation, customize your smoothie with your favorite fruits and vegetables.

Breakfast Meal Prep Tips

Meal preparation can make your mornings easier and guarantee you have a nutritious meal available. Spend a few minutes on Sunday making overnight oats, hard-boiled eggs, and smoothie packets. Keep them in the fridge or freezer for easy assembly throughout the week. This technique saves time and decreases the temptation to skip breakfast or eat less nutritious foods.

Balanced Macronutrients for Morning Energy

Balancing macronutrients in your breakfast is essential for sustaining energy levels and neurological function. Aim for a combination of protein (eggs or Greek yogurt), healthy fats (nuts or avocado), and complex carbohydrates (whole grains or fruits). This balance helps to maintain stable blood sugar levels, provides prolonged energy, and promotes muscle and nerve healing.

Building Balanced Lunch Plates: When putting together a balanced lunch plate, look for a mix of lean meats, healthy fats, complex carbohydrates, and lots of vegetables. Begin with whole grains or leafy greens, then add a serving of lean protein like grilled chicken or tofu, some healthy fats from avocado or almonds, and the rest of your plate with colorful veggies. This balanced approach guarantees that you receive a diverse range of nutrients to fuel your body and keep you content throughout the day.

Salads and soups are great quick and healthful lunches. Make it simple with fresh greens, chopped veggies, grilled prawns or chickpeas, and a delicious dressing. Choose homemade soups that include broth, veggies, and protein sources such as beans or lean meats. Experiment with various herbs and spices to add flavor without increasing calories or sodium. These basic recipes are adaptable, customizable, and ideal for hectic days.

Protein-Packed Lunches: Including protein in your lunch is critical for maintaining energy levels and boosting muscle repair and growth. Choose protein-rich dishes such as grilled salmon, turkey wraps with whole grain tortillas, or quinoa salad with black beans and veggies.

Combine your protein source with substantial carbohydrates such as sweet potatoes or brown grains for sustained energy throughout the afternoon. Make sure to add some healthy fats from sources such as olive oil or avocado to keep you feeling full and satisfied.

Portable Lunch Ideas: When you're on the run, portable lunch options are invaluable. Choose products that can be packed and eaten without utensils, such as whole fruit, cut-up vegetables with hummus, or a handmade trail mix with nuts and dried fruit. Making tiny containers of Greek yogurt or cottage cheese with fruit might also be a convenient and tasty choice. Invest in reusable containers or bento boxes to keep your portable lunches organized and environmentally friendly.

Incorporating Leftovers Creatively: With a little imagination, dinner leftovers can be converted into tasty and filling lunch meals. For a quick and easy lunch, add leftover grilled chicken to salads or stuff it into whole grain wraps. Repurpose roasted veggies by making a robust vegetable stir-fry or blending them into a savory soup. Turn leftover grains into grain bowls with protein, vegetables, and your favorite sauce or dressing. Thinking beyond the box allows you to reduce food waste while still enjoying fascinating new lunch options every day.

Flavorful Supper Recipes for Every Palate: This area has a variety of excellent supper recipes customized to different preferences. These recipes, which range from hearty meat dinners to vegetarian delicacies, are sure to satisfy any appetite. Each dish is carefully developed to maximize flavor so that your meals are not just nutritious but also fulfilling and pleasant.

One-Pot and Sheet Pan foods: Make your supper routine easier by using one-pot and sheet pan foods. These recipes save cleanup while increasing flavor, making them ideal for busy weeknights or leisurely evenings. With only one cooking pot or baking sheet, you can prepare nutritious and tasty meals with little effort.

Plant-Based Supper Options: Discover the world of plant-based dining with our selection of delectable and nutritious supper options. Whether you're a dedicated vegan or simply want to add more plant-based meals to your diet, these dishes are a delightful way to increase your intake of fruits, vegetables, legumes, and grains. Everyone can find something they appreciate, from hearty salads to protein-packed tofu dishes.

solutions for Managing Evening Cravings: Address evening cravings front-on with practical solutions that can help you stay on track with your nutritional goals.

Learn how to detect late-night snacking triggers and find healthier ways to satisfy your needs. You may avoid the temptation to nibble on unhealthy foods and maintain a balanced diet throughout the evening by planning ahead of time and making wise choices.

attentive Eating Practices at Dinner: With simple but effective eating practices, you may transform your dinner experience into one that is attentive and nourishing. Learn to savor each bite, focusing on the flavors, textures, and feelings of your food. Slowing down and being present during dinner might help you digest better, avoid overeating, and develop a deeper appreciation for the food you eat.

Healthy Snacking Habits for Bell's Palsy Management

Treating Bell's Palsy necessitates thoughtful eating habits, including healthy snacking. To improve your overall health, choose low-sugar, high-nutrient snacks.

Concentrate on entire meals such as fruits, vegetables, nuts, and seeds, which contain critical vitamins and minerals needed for healing.

Nutrient-Rich Snack Ideas: Including nutrient-dense snacks in your diet can help with Bell's Palsy management. Consider pairing sliced apples with nut butter, Greek yogurt with berries, or fresh vegetables with hummus. These snacks have a balanced amount of carbohydrates, protein, and healthy fats to help your body repair.

Homemade Snack Recipes: Making your own snacks allows you to have complete control over the ingredients and adjust them to your specific nutritional requirements. Try making energy balls out of oats, almonds, and dates, or bake sweet potato chips seasoned with herbs for a delightful crunch. Experiment with several recipes to find snacks that are both healthy and tasty.

CHAPTER FOUR
Portion Control Tips for Snacking:

Proper portion control is critical for snacking, particularly during Bell's Palsy care. Portion up snacks into tiny dishes or containers rather than consuming them directly from the packet. Focus on the serving sizes recommended by dietary standards to ensure you're getting enough nutrients without going overboard.

Snacks to Manage Cravings and Boost Nutrition: Cravings can derail even the most well-intentioned diet, but picking the right snacks can help manage cravings while also increasing nutrition. Choose foods that satisfy your appetites while supplying essential nutrients.

For example, replace sweet snacks with dark chocolate-covered almonds or satisfy salty cravings with air-popped popcorn sprinkled with nutritional yeast. These options fulfill cravings while also supplying necessary vitamins and minerals to help control Bell's Palsy.

Healthy Snacking Habits for Bell's Palsy Treatment:

Balanced Nutrient Intake: Snacks should include protein, healthy fats, and complex carbs to give long-lasting energy and promote overall health throughout Bell's Palsy rehabilitation.

Fibre Focus: Including fiber-rich foods helps to maintain digestive health, moderate blood sugar levels, and promote fullness, all of which help with weight management.

Hydration Reminder: Incorporate hydrating snacks like fruits and vegetables to stay hydrated, especially during recovery.

Nutrient-Rich Snack Ideas:

Almond Butter and Banana Slices: Spread almond butter on banana slices for a delicious blend of healthy fats, protein, and potassium.

Greek Yoghurt Parfait: A protein-packed, antioxidant-rich snack made by layering Greek yogurt with mixed berries and a sprinkle of almonds.

Steamed edamame sprinkled with sea salt makes a delightful plant-based protein snack.

Avocado bread: For a healthy and tasty snack, top whole-grain bread with mashed avocado, cherry tomatoes, and a drizzle of balsamic glaze.

Hummus & Veggie Sticks: Dip carrots, cucumbers, and bell peppers into hummus for a fiber-rich snack high in vitamins and minerals.

Homemade snack recipes:

Quinoa Salad Cups: Make quinoa salad with chopped veggies and herbs and serve it in lettuce cups for a refreshing and nutritious snack.

Baked Sweet Potato Chips: Slice sweet potatoes thinly, sprinkle with olive oil and your favorite spices, and bake until crispy for a healthier alternative to store-bought chips.

Energy Bites: Combine oats, nut butter, honey, and seeds, then form into bite-sized balls for a quick and energizing snack.

Portion Control Tips for Snacking

Use Smaller Plates or Containers: Choose smaller plates or containers to help limit portion sizes and avoid overeating during snack time.

Pre-portioned Snacks: Divide snacks into individual servings ahead of time to prevent mindless snacking and promote portion control.

Mindful Eating: Pay attention to hunger and fullness cues, and savor each bite to increase satisfaction and avoid overeating.

Snacks to Reduce Cravings and Improve Nutrition:

Dark Chocolate-Covered Almonds: A small serving of dark chocolate-covered almonds is a delightful sweet treat full of antioxidants and healthy fats.

Apple Slices with Cinnamon: Sprinkle cinnamon on apple slices for a naturally sweet and healthful snack that helps control blood sugar levels.

Trail Mix: Combine nuts, seeds, dried fruits, and a sprinkle of dark chocolate chips for a crunchy and filling snack to fulfill cravings.

Meal Plan for a 30-Day Bell's Palsy Management Diet

Week 1:

Day 1-7: Incorporate nutrient-dense foods including lean meats, whole grains, fruits, and vegetables into all meals and snacks.

Week 2:

Day 8-14: Use homemade snacks and recipes from the "Sweet and Savoury Snack Solutions" chapter to promote diversity and healing.

Week 3:

Day 15-21: Experiment with new dishes and snack combinations to make meals more interesting and gratifying.

Week 4:

Prioritise a balanced diet and portion control on Days 22-30 to preserve general health and well-being during recovery. Listen to your body's hunger and fullness cues.

Remember to check with a healthcare practitioner or trained dietitian before making large dietary changes, especially while recovering from disorders such as Bell's Palsy.

Conclusion

Nutrition is critical in the management of Bell's Palsy since it helps with rehabilitation, improves general health, and promotes well-being. The "Bell's Palsy Management Diet Cookbook" was created not only as a collection of recipes but also as a guidance for nourishing the body during this difficult time.

Throughout this cookbook, we've looked at a range of nutrient-dense meals and snacks that give critical vitamins, minerals, and antioxidants needed for healing and maintaining good health. From nourishing soups to tasty salads, and healthful main courses to satisfying snacks, each recipe has been carefully chosen to prioritize both taste and nutrition.

We've emphasized the value of balance, encouraging lean meats, whole grains, healthy fats, and plenty of fruits and vegetables in every meal. Individuals with Bell's Palsy can assist their bodies' natural healing processes by eating a diet rich in these healthful foods while also enjoying delicious and enjoyable meals.

Furthermore, we've included practical recommendations for portion control, mindful eating, and hydration, allowing readers to make informed decisions and create healthy eating habits that will last beyond the pages of this cookbook.

As we come to the end of our culinary adventure together, keep in mind that controlling Bell's Palsy is a multifaceted process that includes not only food modifications but also medical therapy, self-care practices, and emotional support. Individuals with Bell's Palsy can play an active role in their rehabilitation path by fueling their bodies with good foods and adopting a balanced approach to eating.

May this recipe be a great resource and source of inspiration for everyone on the path to wellness while living with Bell's Palsy?

Here's to sustenance, healing, and food's medicinal properties.

THE END